The Muslim Girl's Pocket Guide to Growing Up

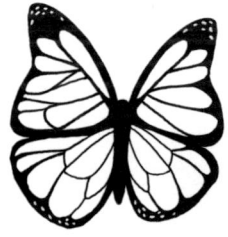

YASMIN EL-HUSARI

Illustrations by Noon Eltoum

The Muslim Girl's Pocket Guide to Growing Up
SBN 978-1-963550-00-9 (paperback edition)

Copyright © 2024 Yasmin El-Husari

Published by Fig & Olive Bookworks, an imprint of Yasmin El-Husari

All rights reserved. No part of this publication may be reproduced, distributed, or transmitted in any form or by any means including photocopying, recording, or other electronic or mechanical methods, without the prior written permission of the publisher.

Cover design and illustrations by Noon Eltoum

Contents

Growing Up	5
Seeing Spots	9
A Hairy Situation	13
Body Safety	19
A Sweaty Dilemma	20
Tahaarah!	22
Periods: The Big Change	25
Periods in Islam	29
Discharge	35
Feminine Protection	38
Bra Measuring Guide	42
Glossary	45

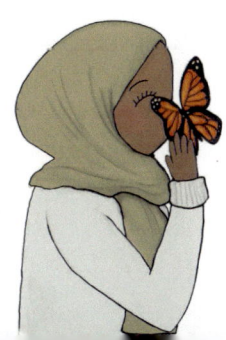

Growing Up

Puberty (Pyoo-ber-tee) is a process of rapid growth that kids go through to become adults. It begins when the **pituitary gland** at the base of the brain sends a signal to the body telling it to start making a special hormone, or chemical. In girls, this hormone is called estrogen. Estrogen is responsible for most of the changes you will see throughout puberty.

Girls usually begin puberty between the ages of 9 and 13 and continue to develop for a few years, until they are 16 or even 20! It's a slow process, and everyone's body has a different timeline. Your genetics, environment, and diet all play a role in determining when this process starts and how fast it goes, so try not to get frustrated. Put your trust in Allah and don't compare yourself to other girls.. Your body will go through puberty at a pace that is right for YOU.

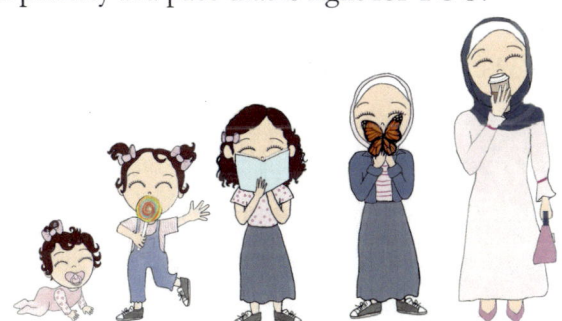

Changes to Expect

Puberty looks a little different for everyone, but there are a few changes you can count on:

- You will grow taller.
- Your body (especially your hips) will become broader.
- You may gain weight.
- Breasts begin to develop.
- You begin to experience strong mood changes.
- Your interests and hobbies may change.
- Your skin may become oily and pimples may develop.
- Your hair may become oily.
- Sweating increases and you will develop body odor.
- You will grow body hair under your arms and between your legs.
- Vaginal discharge begins.
- Periods begin.

The rapid body changes that come with puberty may leave you feeling awkward and clumsy, but it's only temporary. Remember that you are a Muslimah, so stand tall and hold your head high. As strange as some of the points above might sound, they're all part of the natural process of growing up. Keep reading to learn more about what to expect.

*To our Muslim sisters—
with the hope that you will find benefit and inspiration in
these pages.*

*To our families—
may our work always make you proud.*

*To the Islamic Academy of Alabama—
the school that brought together the author and illustrator
so many years ago-
thank you.*

Introduction

> "What good women the womenfolk of the Ansaar were! They did not let shyness prevent them from seeking to understand their religion." – Aishah (ra)

This guide is about growing up. You've done this before. You were once a newborn, then a toddler, and then a child. Now, your body is getting ready for you to become a woman. This stage of life is called puberty, and over the next several years, you will notice major changes in the way you look and feel. It sounds like heavy stuff, but you won't be making this journey alone. Allah (swt) is with you, and practically every woman in the world has traveled this road before.

This book will present scientific facts alongside the majority opinion of Muslim scholars on the various Islamic topics we come upon. You will also find evidence from the Quran and Sunnah throughout the text to support the advice given in these pages. Some topics included here might seem embarrassing, but they're really just a part of life. When you're ready to talk about it, you'll find that trustworthy women in your family can be great sources of information. Read this alone or with a friend, and make use of the glossary at the end to understand the bolded words throughout. See you on the other side!

Ready? Set... Hijab!

"And tell the believing women to lower their gaze and protect their private parts, and not to show off their adornment except what normally appears, and to draw their head coverings over their chests and not to reveal their adornment except to their husbands, or their fathers, or their husband's fathers, or their sons, or their husband's sons, or their brothers or their brother's sons, or their sister's sons, or their fellow women...."
(Quran 24:31)

Hayaa is an Arabic word that refers to modesty, shyness, and healthy shame, all rolled into one. Muslim men and women show *hayaa* when they talk, act, and dress in a decent way that pleases Allah.

A physical part of *hayaa* is awrah, an area of the body that is haram for others to see or touch. Explicit rules of awrah can be found in the Quran and Sunnah.

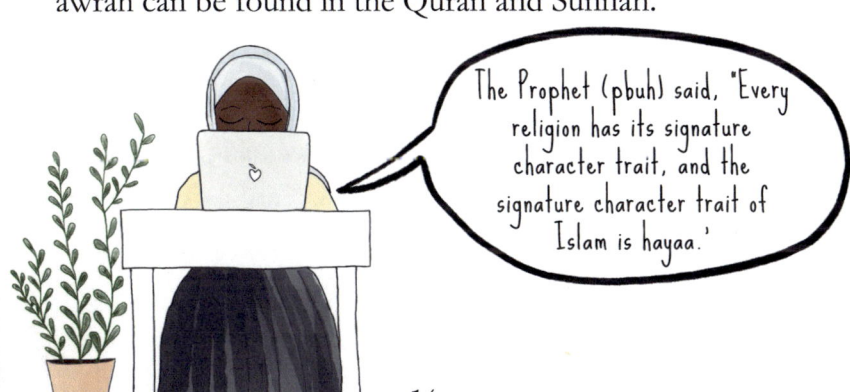

The Prophet (pbuh) said, "Every religion has its signature character trait, and the signature character trait of Islam is hayaa."

A Hairy Situation

Extra sebum production can cause some people to have oily or greasy-looking hair. Knowing your hair type helps guide you when choosing shampoo and other products to keep your hair healthy.

There are three main types of hair:

- **Combination Hair:** Your sebaceous glands are spot on! Your hair has just the right amount of oil.
- **Oily Hair:** Your sebaceous glands are working really well! The extra oil can make your hair look limp and greasy.
- **Dry Hair:** Your sebaceous glands need help making enough oil. Your hair looks fragile and dry.

All hair types are beautiful, but some require a little more care and attention than other types. Learn to love your hair, and be gentle with it. Keep it healthy by avoiding high heat, tight hairstyles, and using chemical treatments like bleaching or hair dye too often. Our body is a gift and an amanah, or trust, from Allah. We are responsible for taking good care of every part of it.

Take Note!

❄ **Diet?** As you grow taller and your body begins to fill out, it is normal and healthy for you to gain weight. You may even notice lines called "stretch marks" on your skin where your skin was forced to stretch in a short amount of time. Adult women have more body fat than young girls. As long as you eat healthy and stay active, whether or not you gain weight during this stage shouldn't be a major concern.

❄ **Need a Bra?** The first signs of breast development are a little soreness and the development of "breast buds," or a small bump under each nipple. This is an exciting sign that it is almost time to buy a training bra! These starter bras are a good place to start until your breasts are big enough for you to size up to a real bra. You can find a bra measuring guide on page 42.

Breasts often continue to develop through the late teen years, so you'll see change over time. A little unevenness in size and shape is normal, even when your breasts are completely developed. It's also important to know that breasts are composed of mainly fat and that their size is determined by genetics, so don't fall for any products that promise to make them bigger.

Taking Life Seriously

> Abu Huraira reported: The Messenger of Allah (pbuh) said, "The first action for which a servant of Allah will be held accountable on the Day of Resurrection will be his prayers. If they are in order, he will have prospered and succeeded. If they are lacking, he will have failed and lost."

Starting puberty is a special milestone in Islam because it means that you've become an adult and are responsible for your own actions. Your shoulder angels have been writing down your good deeds for many years. Once you begin puberty, they'll start recording the bad deeds as well. It can sound scary, but remember that Allah (swt) is the Most Merciful so put your trust in Him. A Muslimah focused on loving and pleasing Allah (swt) will be rewarded with a fulfilling dunya and a beautiful akhirah.

Focus on doing a lot of good deeds, and work on your **salah**. If you weren't taking it seriously before, make sure you practice doing so now. Remember, a strong record of salah means an easy Day of Judgement inshallah.

> Duaa for Help:
> Allahumma a'inni alaa dhikrika, wa shukrika, wa husni 'ibaadatik
>
> "O Allah, help me remember You, to be grateful to You, and to worship You in an excellent manner"

Seeing Spots

If you look very closely in the mirror, you will notice that your face is covered with tiny openings called pores. You have over 5 million pores in your skin all over your body, and these pores allow your skin to breathe and release substances like sweat. Many pores contain a single hair, and under each pore is a small oil producing machine called a **sebaceous gland.** This gland produces an oil called sebum to keep your hair and skin moist and healthy.

Until now, you probably never even noticed sebum production. Puberty changes that. As your body releases a flood of hormones to help regulate puberty, one side effect is that your sebaceous glands will begin to produce extra sebum. When that extra sebum blocks your pores with dead cells, oil, or dirt, your pores can collect bacteria which multiply and cause inflammation. The clogged pore becomes infected and may swell and change color, causing pimples or zits, better known as acne. **Acne** is just a fancy word that means that you have inflamed or irritated pores.

There are four main types of acne:

- **Blackheads**: Open pores that look black because they are clogged by oil and dead skin.
- **Whiteheads:** These pores are also clogged, but in this case, dead skin cells bunch together and cause them to look white.
- **Pimples:** These occur when bacteria attacks clogged pores. White blood cells flood the area to fight infection, giving you a red, pus- filled bump that can be swollen and painful.
- **Cysts:** These are severely inflamed and painful lumps filled with pus. Cystic acne is situated deep in the skin and can cause scarring.

No one chooses to have acne, and getting it is nothing to be ashamed of. The hormone rush that comes with puberty means that nearly everyone will experience breakouts at some point. Severe acne may require a visit to the **dermatologist**, but most of the time acne goes away on its own.

Even adults get acne now and then, so a pimple shouldn't be something that gets in your way. Resist the urge to layer makeup over any breakouts since this can clog your pores and make things even worse. The best way to minimize problems is to wash your face regularly (twice a day) with a mild face wash that works for you.

Don't fall for these common myths!

Acne is only normal if it's on your face...

Acne can appear in many places including the face, neck, back, and chest. That is because our skin is covered in pores that produce sweat and sebum. You should care for non-facial acne just like you do your facial acne. Avoid harsh scrubs or treatment, use antibacterial soaps, acne creams, and moisturizers, and keep affected areas clean by bathing regularly and wearing clean clothes (don't wear that sweaty shirt twice!).

Eating chocolate can cause acne...

Every so often you'll hear someone blame acne on eating fried foods or chocolate or even entire nutrient groups. Your diet can make acne better or worse, but it's generally not going to be the main cause for flair ups. The root cause of acne is hormonal, and scientists have never been able to pinpoint specific acne-causing foods because different bodies have different sensitivity levels. The general rule is to eat a varied diet that focuses on whole foods. There's nothing wrong with some chocolate every once in a while.

Washing your face often can prevent breakouts...

Bad bacteria definitely makes acne breakouts worse, but again, the main cause of acne is your hormones. Be patient. Using face wash too often can cause dryness, and the skin often reacts by increasing oil production and making acne worse. Using face wash twice a day (morning and evening) is more than enough, and there's no need to use harsh scrubs. Instead, reduce the introduction of bacteria to your face. Wash your hands before touching your face and make sure that surfaces like your phone screen are cleaned often.

You should never, ever pop a pimple...

It is true that popping a pimple can push bacteria under the skin and cause a scar or pit. However, there are times when you can (gently!) extract blackheads and whiteheads to help them heal. Just remember to use clean hands, never use your nails, and always make sure the pimple is ready before you

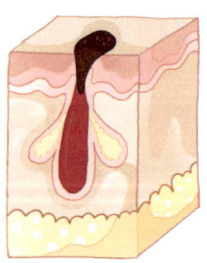

attempt to pop it. If you have to force it, it's probably too early. When in doubt, it is better to leave it alone to reduce the risk of permanent scarring. Acne generally heals on its own within a couple of weeks.

There are different levels of awrah, the most private being the area from the belly button to the knees. Except in the case of a necessary medical situation, no one, not even your mom, should see or touch this area. No one should ask to see your awrah, and you shouldn't see anyone else's either.

Once we are old enough to clean and care for our own bodies, the rules of awrah apply to both what we show from our own bodies and what we see from others. The rule extends to nonMuslims, so practice lowering your eyes, even when watching a screen or in a public area. And although awrah applies when others are around, you should also avoid unnecessary nakedness when you are alone.

Puberty expands your awrah to cover more of your body, but the rules of what to cover change depending on who is in the room. The basic categories you should remember are:

- **Among Muslim women:** Your awrah is the area between your belly button and your knees. This means you can wear anything you want as long as it's not skin-tight, see-through, or above the knee. There is no such thing as too modest though!

**Note that once a girl begins to wear hijab, she should only take it off in front of trustworthy people who won't talk about what they see. Muslimahs never describe other women's hair or bodies to men.

Men are divided into two categories, mahram and nonMahram. A mahram is a man whom Allah (swt) has permanently forbidden you from marrying. This includes men like your father, your grandfathers, and your parents' brothers. You can find a full graphic at the back of this book.

With Mahram Men: You don't have to wear hijab in front of them, but your awrah extends from at least your chest to your knees.

With Non-Mahram Men: Once you start to show major signs of puberty, your awrah is everything except for your face and hands. It's time to start wearing hijab!

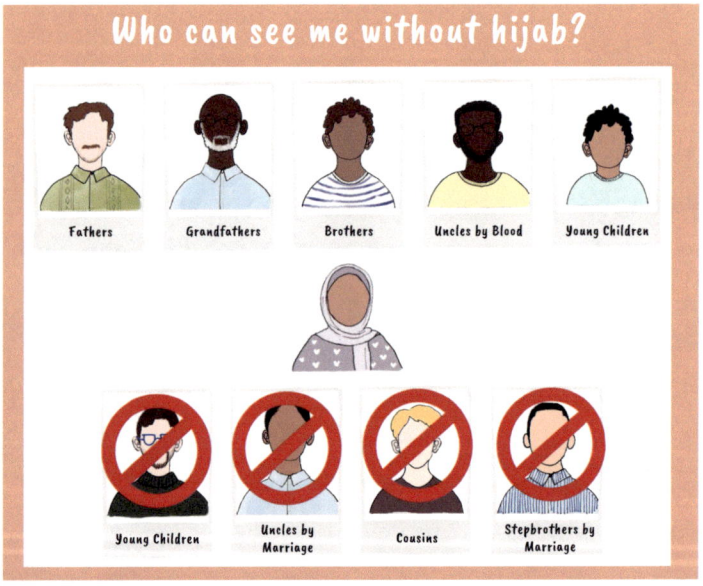

Hijab is *Ibadah*

"O Prophet! Tell your wives and your daughters and the women of the believers to draw their outer cloaks over their bodies. That will be better, that they should be recognized and not hurt. And Allah is Ever Oft-Forgiving, Most Merciful." (Quran 33:59)

Allah (swt) is our Creator. Everything good in our lives comes from Him, and everything we struggle with is a test of our faith and a way to get closer to Him. Allah (swt) blessed us with beauty, and He ordered us to cover that beauty with hijab. Just like the **sahabiyat** obeyed the order of hijab immediately after they heard it, we obey because we love Allah (swt) and we want to please Him. He (swt) promised us a great reward for all of our struggles for His sake.

With that being said, it won't always be easy. True hijab covers us from head to toe and can make us stand out where it might be easier to fit in. Wearing hijab is a form of worship that can strengthen our faith. We might not feel very confident when we start, but by becoming "visible Muslimahs," we practice speaking up for our faith and learn to be proud of our Islam.

Conditions for Hijab

- Cover everything except for the hands and face— no hair, ears, or neck should show
- Loose outfits— Nothing tight or see-through
- Sleeves should reach your wrists (don't pull them up!)
- Legs should be covered to the ankles
- Most scholars say that the feet should be covered
- Accessories like anklets and earrings should not show, but rings are okay
- No makeup (cover your beauty!)
- Avoid noisy jewelry like armfuls of bangles as well as shoes that draw attention to your movements
- Avoid strong perfume or other long-lasting scents
- Avoid using accessories that add volume above the head (e.g. large hair donuts)

Our beauty is a gift from Allah (swt), and the best way to thank Him is to use it in a way that pleases Him. The list above may seem restrictive, but remember that Muslim women do not wear hijab all the time. Many of the above items like wearing perfume and makeup are halal when in private among women or among mahram men at home.

Body Safety

The rules of awrah and hijab are great ways to define your personal space. Unless there is an emergency or medical reason, nonMahram men and women should never touch, not even to shake hands. Here are some other body safety rules to be aware of:

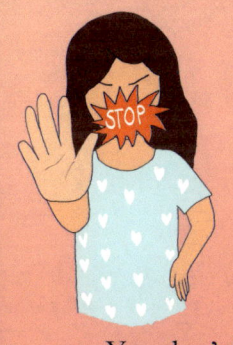

- NEVER, EVER take pictures of yourself with your awrah uncovered. Any images that make it to the internet are permanent.
- Practice saying "no" loudly and clearly. No one, not even an adult, has the right to touch you or make you touch them in a way that feels uncomfortable.
- You don't have to keep anyone's secrets. Speak up if something feels wrong.
- Do not share pictures or private information like your birthdate or address with strangers online.
- Never do or say anything on videochat that you wouldn't do or say in person.
- Tell a trusted adult if anyone ever tries to threaten you in person or online. That is the best way to get help.
- Respect the body safety of others (treat others like you would want to be treated).

A Sweaty Dilemma

Your sebaceous glands aren't the only organ activated by puberty. Your sweat glands will start to work overtime too. You may notice yourself sweating when you're hot, tired, stressed, or sometimes, seemingly for no reason at all.

> "Truly, Allah loves those who turn to Him constantly and He loves those who keep themselves clean and pure." (Quran, 2:222).

Humans have two kinds of sweat glands:

- **Eccrine glands** cover your entire body except for your lips and ears. Ever since you were a baby, they've produced clear, odorless perspiration, or sweat, to help cool you off.

- **Apocrine glands** (many located in your armpits) begin working when you hit puberty. They produce a sweat that bacteria love to munch on. The breakdown of this sweat causes an onion-like body odor, or B.O, that can cling to your skin and clothes.

Pay close attention to how you smell and work on your personal care. A Muslimah always does her best to smell squeaky clean!

There are two primary products that can be used to control underarm odor:

- **Deodorant** covers up odors with a fragrance and helps you smell better.
- **Antiperspirant** blocks the pores to reduce the amount of sweat produced; can also carry a fragrance

Both types of products should be applied to clean, dry skin for best results. Do some research and consult with a trusted adult before deciding on which to use. A trip to the store or pharmacy will introduce you to a multitude of products. Your options range from natural to chemical to roll-ons to sprays and more, and there are many scents to choose from (although unscented is also an option). Read the instructions before applying any product, and watch for any allergic reactions.

First Thing's First... The first step to smelling fresh is to reduce the amount of bacteria on your skin. A daily shower and clean change of clothes before applying any product is the way to go. Also consider carrying an extra shirt and deodorant to school. If you start to smell funny during the day, you can always step into a bathroom stall and clean up with a soapy paper towel, reapply deodorant, and change your shirt to freshen up. It will take effort at first, but you'll get the hang of it soon enough.

Tahaarah!

> The Prophet (pbuh) said, "Ten are the practices of fitrah: . . . using the siwaak, snuffing water up the nose, cutting the nails, washing the finger joints, plucking the hair under the armpits, shaving the pubic hairs and cleaning one's private parts with water." The narrator said: 'I have forgotten the tenth, but it may have been rinsing the mouth.'

Sunan of Fitrah

Cleanliness is a part of faith. Although the above mentioned are all important sunnahs, we will focus on a few for the purpose of this book.

1. Nail Care

Long painted nails may be fashionable, but our **deen** teaches us to keep them short. This prevents the accumulation of dirt and bacteria under the nail bed. The Prophet (pbuh) used to cut his nails once a week before Jumah. We also need bare nails when making wudu for water to reach our nails. Don't worry though. There are days when women are excused from salah and can wear nail polish all day. We will get to that in a bit.

> "He set a time for us to trim our moustaches, cut our nails, pluck our armpit hair and shave our pubic hair; we were not to leave that for more than forty days."
> -Anas bin Malik about the Prophet (pbuh)

2. Armpit Hair

A combination of sweat and underarm hair can pack a hard punch of BO. The **sunnah** for both men and women is to pull the hair out by the root, although shaving is also a viable option. If you decide to pull the hair out, you can choose between waxes, tweezers, or even epilators (motorized hair removers). It can hurt a little at first, but if you trim the hair short before you start and remove it regularly, it will become less and less painful over time.

3. Pubic Hair

Pubic hair refers to the hair that will start growing in the "bikini area" between your legs. It will eventually become dense and coarse. Having pubic hair is an important development because it is a clear sign that you are officially an adult under Islamic law. And although pubic hair is completely natural, the sunnah is to remove it. Your options for this include using razors, hair removal creams, or even wax if you do it yourself.

If you decide to use a razor, use one designed for the pubic area and trim your pubic hair short before you start. Use a shaving cream and exfoliate before and after to prevent ingrown hairs. Never share your razor, and replace it often to avoid shaving with a dull blade. You can ask an adult for other tips, but keep the rules of awrah in mind!

Keep your pubic hair short enough prevent the accumulation of impurities, sweat, or dirt that can lead to irritation or infection. Forty days is the longest you can wait between shaves, but it is best to tend to the hair before it gets too long.

4. Visiting the Bathroom

Alhamdulillah as Muslims, we are guided even when it comes to what to do in the bathroom:

- Sit or squat; do not stand while urinating.
- Do not speak while using the toilet.
- It is sunnah and highly preferred to wash your private parts with water using your left hand each time.
- If water is unavailable and you use tissues, wipe an odd number of times (at least three).
- Wipe front to back, **not** back to front to prevent fecal bacteria from entering the urinary tract.
- Take care to prevent **najasa** from contaminating your clothing.

Periods: The Big Change

Women usually experience a **period** once a month, and it is when some fluid, including blood, exits the body from the **vagina** (one of the openings between the legs). Sounds scary, but the actual release of fluid shouldn't hurt. Much of the time, you'll hardly feel it. Most girls get their first period between the ages of 9 to 15, about 2 years after they develop breasts. Genetics, diet, and environment are the major deciding factors for when you get your first period; everyone has their own "right time."

Getting a monthly period is probably the biggest change that girls expect from puberty. Although getting your first period can be a bit surprising, it's no cause for worry. This is a very natural process, and it indicates that your body is healthy and working properly.

Why do we have periods in the first place?

Only women get periods, and they are part of a bigger phenomenon called the **menstrual cycle**. This is a 23 to 35 day process that the female body goes through every month to enable it to have babies. The most visible part of the menstrual cycle is the period, but there is actually so much more going on behind the scenes. Take a look:

The Menstrual Cycle

1 Girls are born with two almond-sized **ovaries** which contain thousands of eggs. When you reach puberty, the hormone estrogen tells an ovary to release an egg. The ovaries generally take turns releasing only one egg every month.

2 The released egg takes a two week trip along the **fallopian tube** from the ovaries towards the uterus.

3 The **uterus** is a hollow organ the size of your fist. This is where babies grow. A hormone called progesterone signals the walls of the uterus to thicken with a soft lining of blood and tissue. If the egg is fertilized by a male **sperm**, it will settle in this lining and grow until it becomes a baby.

4 Most of the time, the egg is not fertilized and the lining of the uterus is not needed. Therefore, it dissolves and leaves the body through the **vagina** as a reddish fluid widely known as the period.

Menstruation: (aka having periods) The uterus discharges a reddish (or sometimes brown) fluid containing blood and the uterine lining.

It is very common for girls who just started their menstrual cycles to have irregular periods. At the beginning, your period could last for one day or for ten, and it could come every month or once every few. You might also find that your periods are lighter or heavier than that of your friends. No two women are the same, and your body is trying to find a rhythm specific to you. It is normal for girls to take two years or more to settle into a dependable cycle.

Pre-Menstrual Syndrome (PMS): This is the name of the symptoms that a girl may begin to experience 1 to 14 days before she gets her period. These symptoms can be physical or emotional and can include conditions such as moodiness or sadness, back aches, sore breasts, cravings, bloating, insomnia or difficulty sleeping, and headaches.

**Extreme symptoms that interfere with your ability to carry out daily activities every month may be a sign of a medical problem. Your regular doctor may refer you to a specialist called a gynecologist to find a cause for your symptoms.

> It may look like a lot, but the average woman only loses about 70 ml (or a few teaspoons) of fluid during her period, and only about half of that is blood. You can still do the things you normally do like exercising, showering, and eating your favorite foods while menstruating. Most people will not know that you are on your period unless you tell them.

Cramps: An extremely common symptom women experience with PMS is "period cramps" which feels like an ache in the lower back or abdomen or along the inner thighs.

During a period, the uterus contracts to push out menstrual blood. If it contracts too strongly, the uterus can press against nearby blood vessels, cutting off the oxygen supply to its muscle tissue and causing pain, or cramps. You can sooth persistent cramps with a warm bath, a heating pad held over your lower stomach, or exercise (lack of exercise has actually been linked to painful menstrual cramps). If cramps become a serious problem, ask a trusted adult about pain relievers.

 **PMS symptoms can persist for quite a few days into the period. Sleeping well, eating healthy foods, getting regular exercise, and getting necessary vitamins and minerals throughout the month are all ways to help control PMS symptoms and make them more manageable.

Periods in Islam

You are excused from two major forms of **ibadah** while on your period: salah and fasting. You also should not touch the **mus'haf** with your bare hand during this time. You don't need to make up prayers that you missed during your period, but you should make up any days of missed Ramadan fasts before next Ramadan.

When Do I Stop Praying?

You should stop praying when you see either blood or dark brown discharge in your underwear at your time of the month. If you are fasting, you should also break your fast. If it is salah time but you haven't managed to pray it yet, make a note of it. You will make it up when you can pray again.

Just because you can't pray doesn't mean that you should cut off all forms of worship during your period. That can make it hard to get back on track once it's over. Stay connected to Allah by reciting Quran from memory and from digital devices. This is also good chance to work on making Duaa and Thikr as well as seeking Islamic knowledge through books or lectures.

When Can I Start Praying Again?

Periods last between two to seven days although some women bleed for longer than ten. You'll know that your period is over when you see white or clear discharge or when you have become completely dry.

It is worth noting that menstrual flow is not continuous as you can go hours without bleeding before restarting again. Women generally experience the heaviest flow in the first two or three days of the period. You'll likely be able to feel a "gush" of fluids during these days. The bleeding then slows to spotting or colored discharge until it finally stops completely at the end of the period. Again, normal is what your body decides is normal for you. When in doubt, make a note of the prayer time and wait for a few hours. Once you are sure your period is over, it is time to make **ghusl**.

> Once your body gets into a consistent routine, you will know how long your periods normally last. If you happen to have an unusually long period or a period that stops then starts again <u>outside of what is normal for you</u>, this blood is called istihaada or "other blood." You should continue to pray, but make wudu before each salah and make sure that your underwear is clean.

Making Ghusl

Ghusl is the term used for the ritual bath that purifies major **najasa**. It is important for both men and women to learn it properly because it directly affects the validity of salah. We must make ghusl at the end of our periods and after the release of maniy. The steps of ghusl can be divided into two categories: **fard** and **sunnah**.

There are two fard requirements for ghusl to count so that you can begin praying again:

- **Making an intention before you start.** This means that you should go into the bath or shower mindfully, aware that you are about to make ghusl (you don't have to say any special words though).

- **Allowing water to reach the entire body.** This includes the inside of your ears and all the way down to your scalp.

If you ever forget the full procedure of ghusl or find yourself short on time, fulfilling these two requirements is enough for you to be pure and able to pray.

Once you have the fard covered, you can move on to learning the steps of ghusl to get rewarded for doing things like the Prophet (pbuh) did.

Steps of Ghusl

1. Make your intention and say bismillah.
2. Wash your hands three times.
3. Use your left hand to wash away all impurities from your private parts.
4. Make wudu like you normally would.
5. Pour water on your head (or stand under the shower), allowing it to reach your scalp, three times. Be sure to rub the water in.
6. Wash the right, then left side of your body, making sure there are no dry spots.

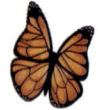

If you tend to wear your hair in a style with lots of braids, you do not have to take your braids out every time you make ghusl. You do, however, need to pour water over your head three times and take special care to ensure that water reaches your entire scalp.

Once you've made ghusl, so long as you haven't done anything that would normally break your wudu like passing gas or using the restroom, you can consider yourself on wudu and begin praying. Don't forget to make up the prayer you missed when you first got your period.

❀ It is very important to know when your period ends. If your period ends before Fajr athan during Ramadan, then you are required to fast that day, even if you didn't manage to make ghusl until after the end of Fajr time.

Tips for the Last Day of Your Period

- Change often. It is easier to identify the end of your period with a clean pad.
- Visit the bathroom frequently and note the prayer time when you last noticed a spot.
- Delay ghusl until the last half hour before the next athan to confirm without missing a prayer time.
- If you're not sure when exactly your period ended, make up an extra prayer, just in case it ended earlier than you noticed.
- If you spot after making ghusl and praying, try not to get frustrated. Repeat the ghusl when you are more sure.
- When in doubt, WAIT.

Examples

- Fatimah got her period right after Thuhr Athan on Monday before she had a chance to pray it. She made sure to mark that prayer on her calendar. Her period ended at Thuhr the next Monday, but since she was at school, she did not get to make ghusl until Asr time. Fatimah is required to pray Thuhr from the day she got her period, and she should also pray Thuhr and Asr from the day her period ended.

- Saleemah took a shower when she got home from school to refresh after a hot day. She realized a few hours later that her period must have ended before she took her shower. She should still make ghusl before beginning salah because she did not intend to make ghusl when she showered.

- Maryam woke up after Fajr and realized that her period must have ended some time last night. She should pray Isha and Fajr before continuing about her day.

- It is Ramadan and Layla went into the bathroom ten minutes before Maghrib to make wudu. She noticed that she got her period. She should break her fast immediately and mark that day to make up. She is excused from all prayers including taraweeh until her period is over.

Vaginal Discharge

The vagina is a self-lubricating organ. Just like your mouth needs saliva to stay moist and your nose uses mucus to trap dust and other particles, your vagina also contains fluids to keep it clean and to get rid of any infection-causing bad bacteria. That means that even between periods, you will often notice **vaginal discharge** in your underwear. This is a fluid made up of mostly cells and bacteria, and it ranges in color from clear to light brown, depending on where you are in your menstrual cycle. Vaginal discharge will also range in thickness and consistency throughout the month, so don't be alarmed if it doesn't look the same all the time. You will have discharge for most of your adult life.

Make sure that you wash yourself with water and dry your **genitals** completely every time you go to the bathroom or take a shower. Avoid using any scented products in your genital area, even if the products are advertised to be safe. The vagina is self-cleaning, so using water to wash away visible impurities is enough. Soaps and other products can affect the **pH** of a healthy vagina and cause an infection.

Islamic law recognizes multiple types of vaginal discharge, and it also gives us guidelines on how to deal with them. It will take a bit of practice, but you will soon be able to recognize the different types and deal with them effortlessly.

- **Rutooba:** This discharge is a wetness that is constantly present in the vagina. It can be in varying levels of stickiness depending on the time of your cycle. Um Atiyah, a Sahabiyah once said, "After Tuhr (being clean from our periods) we would not consider discharge anything." Therefore, there is no need to renew wudu if this is the discharge you are experiencing.
- **Wadi:** At times, your body releases a cloudy or clear discharge after you urinate. Take your time when cleaning yourself and standing up after using the toilet because this type of discharge is *najis,* or ritually impure. Getting it on your clothes means they need to be changed and washed.
- **Mathi:** This type of discharge is triggered by thoughts of the opposite sex. Sometimes consuming romantic movies or literature or even just having romantic thoughts can cause funny feelings and secretion of discharge into your underwear. This discharge is najis and breaks your wudu. It must be washed off your clothes and body before you can pray

- **Maniy**: Thin white or yellowish discharge that the body releases unintentionally after a dream or intentionally after heightened sexual pleasure. This discharge leads to a state of ritual impurity called **janaabah**. You must wash it off your clothes and make ghusl before praying or reciting Quran.

Discharge is normal. However, if it smells fishy, looks gray, green, or clumpy like cottage cheese, or you start feeling burning or itchiness in your genitals, you may have bacterial vaginosis or a yeast infection. Experiencing sharp pain when you urinate could also be a sign of a urinary tract infection, or UTI. These conditions are very common, and they don't necessarily mean that you did anything wrong. Something as simple as being stressed or taking antibiotics can be the cause

Don't be afraid to tell a trusted adult if you are experiencing these symptoms. Although it can feel embarrassing to talk about these conditions, ignoring infections doesn't make them go away. Untreated, some of these can lead to more serious health issues.

Muslims are encouraged to seek medical care when they need it. Doctors and nurses are trained to help you without compromising your shyness. Often, a simple prescription cream is all it takes to make you feel better.

Feminine Hygiene Products

Feminine hygiene products are products used to absorb fluids from your period and to keep you feeling clean at other times of the month.

During Your Period

The main product you will use during your period is a "pad," which is basically a cloth pad with a sticky backing worn inside of your underwear. This can be found at any pharmacy or grocery store. Depending on your body type and how heavy your flow is every month, you can choose between different lengths, widths, and levels of absorbancy, as well as between different brands. Many of them have "wings," which are just tabs on the side that wrap around the outside of your underwear to hold them in place and keep them from slipping around.

You may decide to opt for more natural options or choose to use reusable cloth pads or period underwear. Some women even have different types of pads on hand for different stages of their period, or wear thicker pads at night to prevent leaking. Period protection can be as simple or as complicated as you want it to be. The possibilities are endless!

Although many pads guarantee up to eight hours of protection, don't wait that long between changes. Refresh your pad regularly throughout the day to avoid leaks and bad smells. If you aren't bleeding enough to fill a pad even after many hours, consider switching to a thinner one or even to a pantiliner that better fits your flow.

Other popular period products are tampons and menstrual cups. Unlike pads which catch menstrual fluid as it leaves the body, these are inserted inside the vagina to capture menstrual flow from within. Women prefer them for situations like swimming or when wearing tighter clothing that would reveal the shape of a pad.

Internal protection is not haram, but many traditional cultures seriously frown on using it. Additionally, these products can introduce harmful chemicals into the vaginal canal and create an environment for bacteria to multiply and cause infections. In extreme cases, leaving tampons in for too long can lead to a serious condition called toxic shock syndrome, or TSS. It is best to start with pads and consult with a trusted Muslim adult before deciding to branch out.

Most women buy some form of feminine protection every month, so don't feel shy about getting what you need. You can always turn to your mother or an older sister for help if you feel uncomfortable.

When You're Done

Each package of pads contains instructions on how to both put them on and dispose of them properly. Feminine hygiene products should never go in the toilet because they can clog up the plumbing. You should also never leave a used pad open in the trash for others to see or smell. Be courteous. Wrap the used protection well so that it doesn't draw attention (you can use toilet paper to do so if needed). Most public restrooms provide a closed-lid trash can in each stall for easy disposal of period products. Before you leave the bathroom, make sure that no trace of your period is left on or in the toilet.

Liners for in Between

It can be a hassle to deal with discharge, especially when it comes to the kind you have to clean off your clothes before you pray. That is where "pantiliners" come in. These are smaller, thinner pads that are worn on the inside of your underwear when your menstrual flow is super light or just day-to-day to help you manage discharge and feel clean.

Although you should still be changing your underwear regularly, you can manage discharge throughout the day by simply changing pantiliners rather than underwear. Just like pads, pantiliners come in a variety of brands, sizes, and styles. Shop around and find the perfect one for you.

Be Prepared

You might not know when you'll get your first period, but you can still be prepared. It's a good idea to keep a clean pair of underwear and a pad in makeup bag in your backpack or locker at school. If you don't have a pad, you can use a wad of tissues as a temporary solution. School nurses usually carry feminine hygiene products with their supplies, or you can turn to a trusted female teacher or staff member for help. Sometimes, a friend may even be carrying an extra and would be happy to lend you what you need!

Once you get home, any stains in your underwear can be washed out easily by hand with cold water and some soap before going into the laundry.

Get into the habit of marking your period start and end dates on a calendar, and make a note of any missed fasts or prayers. This will help you predict the date of your next period as well as keep track of any deeds you have to make up. You can also download a free period tracking app on a phone or tablet to do the same thing. Be sure to make a note of your Ramadan fasts as you make them up. You want to finish fasting all of your missed days before the next Ramadan rolls around.

Bra Measuring Guide

Your breast size and shape will change throughout your lifetime, so make it a habit to measure yourself before bra-shopping trips to get a good fit. You can use string or yarn to measure in place of measuring tape.

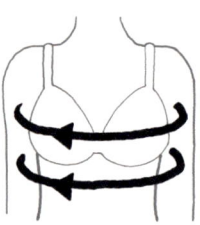

1. Wrap a measuring tape around your ribcage just under your breasts where your bra band would sit. Make sure the tape is level. If you get an odd number, add five inches. If you get an even number, add four. This is your band size.

2. Measure around your torso at the fullest part of your breasts at nipple level. Make sure it's not too tight.

3. Find the difference between the two numbers and refer to the table to find your cup size.

Difference	Cup Size
0	AA
1 inch	A
2 inches	B
3 Inches	C
4 Inches	D

You may get a slightly different fit when switching between brands or styles of bras. Don't be afraid to shop around until you find what works for you.

Example: Sarah's first measurement was 27 inches. She added 5 inches to get a band size of 32. Her second measurement was 33 inches. 33 minus 32 is 1, so Sarah needs an A cup. Her current size is 32A.

WHO CAN SEE ME WITHOUT HIJAB?

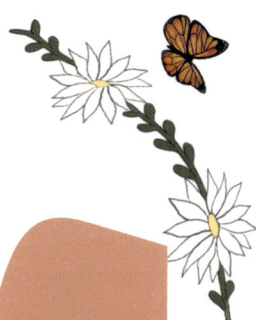
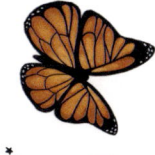

Mahram Men
- Father
- Stepfathers
- Grandfathers
- Brothers by blood
- Uncles by blood*
- Milk Brothers**

Women & Children
- Trustworthy Muslim women
- Trustworthy nonMuslim women
- Young children

In the Future...
- Husband
- Father-in-law
- Sons
- Nephews
- Husband's sons
- Son-in-laws

*Uncles by marriage are NOT considered mahram
**Milk siblings nursed from the same woman at least five times before the age of weaning.

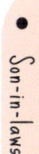
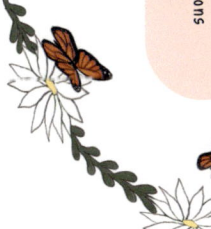

A Note from the Author

My dear sister, thank you for letting me be your guide. The changes mentioned in this book may seem daunting, but there is so much joy to be found in your teenage years. You will struggle as you get used to your new body and learn how to care for it. That much is true. But every conquered challenge will give you new confidence as both your body and mind mature.

Every adult has once been in your shoes, so be patient and take heart. Don't compare yourself too much to those around you. Allah (swt) created us in so many beautiful shapes, sizes, and variations, so learn to be content with what you were given. Remember to say "Alhamdulillah" when you look in the mirror. Your teenage years are a journey, not your destination. Enjoy them, and focus on what will truly matter in the end.

The most important thing is to take care of yourself. Set goals, adopt beneficial habits, explore your interests, and seek knowledge that will help you become who you want to be as an adult. Use your time wisely and build a strong relationship with Allah (swt) so that your heart can find peace in this life and the next.

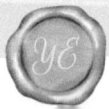

Glossary

Body odor: an unpleasant smell that can result from the mixing of bacteria and perspiration

Deen: Arabic for religion or way of life

Dermatologist: a doctor who specializes in the largest organ in the body, the skin

Estrogen: a female hormone produced by the ovaries that is responsible for producing and maintaining female characteristics

Fallopian tubes: tubes that connect the two ovaries to the uterus

Fard: action required and rewarded by Allah. Not completing it is considered a sin.

Hadith: teachings and sayings of the Prophet Muhammad (pbuh)

Hormones: chemical messengers released by glands that help control functions that occur inside the body

Ibadah: the Arabic word for worship, and it includes all actions that Allah (swt) loves

Istihaadah: vaginal bleeding that occurs outside of the timing of the period

Janaabah: a state of ritual impurity that results from the release of maniy

Genitals: the external reproductive organs in the pubic area

Ghusl: the Islamic ritual bath required to purify major impurities

Maniy: discharge that results from sexual climax or wet dreams and requires ghusl for purification

Mathi: discharge that results from sexual feelings without climax and requires wudu and purification of clothing

Menstrual cycle: the time measured from the start of one period to the start of the next

Menstruation: also known as the period, the monthly shedding of the inner lining of the uterus through the vagina

Mus'haf: the Quran printed and bound into a physical book

Najasa: the Islamic term for ritual impurity which must be removed to pray

Ovaries: two almond sized organs that contain a woman's egg cells and produce the hormones estrogen and progesterone

(pbuh): acronym for "peace be upon him"

pH: a scale used to measure how acidic or basic something is

Pituitary gland: a pea shaped organ found at the base of your brain responsible for producing important hormones

Progesterone: a female hormone that causes the lining of the uterus to thicken in preparation for receiving the egg cell.

Puberty: the teen years when a child's body begins to change into that of an adult's

Rutooba: Vaginal discharge that is generally present in the body. Does not require any special purification.

Salah: the five daily prayers at prescribed times. One of the basic pillars of Islam.

Sperm: the male reproductive cell

Sahabiyah: a girl or woman who met the Prophet (pbuh) and accepted Islam during his lifetime

Sebaceous gland: an organ that secretes oils through hair follicles to lubricate hair and skin

Sunan al- Fitrah: sunnah actions that have to do with true human nature. They are highly recommended actions to engage in.

Sunnah: teaching, sayings, and life example of the Prophet Muhammad (pbuh)

(swt): acronym for Subhanahu wa Ta'ala, Arabic for "may He be glorified and exalted"

Uterus: the female organ lined with soft tissue where an egg is nourished into a baby

Vagina: the muscular passage that leads from the uterus to the outside of the body

Wathi: Discharge sometimes released after urination

About the Author

Yasmin El-Husari is a high school teacher currently working on her master's in instructional design. She has been involved in halaqas and Quranic education for over 10 years. She wrote the first version of this pocket guide during her freshman year of college. The book you hold in your hands is the fruit of years of research, learning, and teaching.

About the Illustrator

Noon Eltoum MD, MPH, a lifelong friend and sister of the author, is a doctor and researcher who loves to paint and draw. Her art journey started on Instagram in 2020 with her page "The Confluence" where she showcases her artwork. Illustrating a book she herself benefited from as a young Muslimah is an honor and a dream come true.

Made in the USA
Columbia, SC
12 March 2024